The Weight Loss Code: Sure Tips For Natural Weight Loss

By

Gregory William

Table of contents

Introduction

In recent years, low-carbohydrate diets have gained popularity as a means of shedding pounds and enhancing general health. The idea is straightforward: consume fewer carbohydrates, the body's main source of energy, and rely more on protein and fat. Weight loss, better blood sugar regulation, less inflammation, and enhanced cardiovascular health are just a few advantages that may result from this change in macronutrient balance.

However, because there are so many variants and viewpoints on what defines a "low-carb" diet, the low-carbohydrate diet may also be complicated subject to understand. Some specialists advise completely avoiding all carbohydrates, while others advocate a more reasonable strategy that still permits a small quantity of carbohydrates in the diet. Because of this, it may be challenging for people to choose the strategy that would work best for them and to figure out how to apply it in a satisfying manner.

This book, which strives to offer a thorough overview of the low-carbohydrate diet, including its possible advantages and disadvantages as well as the most recent scientific studies on the subject, fills that need. It will examine the many low-carb eating plans and assist you in selecting the strategy that may work finest for your particular requirements and objectives. Additionally, it offers helpful pointers and guidance on how to carry out the diet, such as meal plans and recipes, as well as methods for overcoming typical obstacles and maintaining the diet over the long term.

This book will give you the information and resources you need to successfully adopt a low-carbohydrate diet and meet your health and wellness goals, whether you're an experienced low-carb dieter or you're just beginning to investigate the idea. Let's explore the various advantages of this ground-breaking strategy for nutrition now.

Chapter One

What exactly is a low-carb diet?

A low-carb diet limits the consumption of carbs, which are often found in meals like bread, pasta, and sugar, and instead emphasizes foods that are high in protein and good fats. A low-carb diet aims to reduce the consumption of foods that boost blood sugar levels and insulin production because they are readily converted to sugar and absorbed into the bloodstream. In order to maintain stable blood sugar levels and consume fewer calories overall, persons on low-carb diets seek to eat more whole, unprocessed foods that are slowly digested.

How Can a Low-Carbohydrate Diet Help You Lose Weight?

A low-carbohydrate diet's main tenet is that it forces the body to burn fat for energy instead of glucose (sugar). When the body burns fat, weight loss happens. When the body cannot get enough carbohydrates, it must get its energy from fat reserves, which causes weight loss.

Additionally, because insulin is a hormone that encourages hunger, the low insulin levels linked to a low-carb diet may cause a decrease in total caloric consumption. People on low-carb diets may find it simpler to manage their calorie intake and maintain their diet objectives by decreasing insulin production.

Diets Low in Carbohydrates Promote Weight Loss

Promotes fat loss: A low-carb diet can result in significant fat loss by limiting carbohydrate intake and motivating the body to burn fat for energy.

Reduces insulin levels and improves insulin sensitivity: By reducing the consumption of high-carbohydrate meals, a low-carbohydrate diet can reduce insulin levels and increase insulin sensitivity, which will result in better weight loss outcomes.

Energy levels can rise when the body uses fat as fuel rather than carbohydrates, which can also have a positive impact on general well-being.

Can enhance heart health: By lowering the risk of high blood pressure, high cholesterol, and other related health issues, a low-carbohydrate diet can promote heart health by restricting the consumption of processed and high-carbohydrate foods.

Concerns and Potential Risks of a Low-Carbohydrate Diet

Deficiencies in some nutrients can develop over time on a low-carb diet since it limits the consumption of fiber and certain vitamins and minerals, among other essential elements.

Sticking to the diet can be taxing and restricting, which is why some people find it hard to maintain a low-carb diet over the long haul.

When carbs are limited, people may feel tempted to consume more protein and fat, which can result in overeating and a high intake of undesirable saturated fats.

A low-carb diet might not be suitable for everyone, particularly those with diabetes, liver illness, renal disease, or other medical issues. Before beginning a low-carb diet, people with these diseases should speak with their doctor.

In conclusion, a low-carb diet can be a successful means of encouraging weight reduction and enhancing general health, but it's crucial to approach the diet in a balanced and informed manner, taking into account specific demands and medical circumstances. It's always better to seek specific advice from a physician or a qualified dietitian before beginning a low-carbohydrate diet.

Chapter Two

Knowing Carbohydrates and How They Affect Weight Loss

What exactly are carbs?

One kind of macronutrient that gives the body energy is carbohydrates. They can be present in a wide range of foods, such as cereals, fruits, vegetables, and sweets. Glucose, a product of the breakdown of carbohydrates, is used by the body as an energy source.

There are two primary categories of carbohydrates: simple and complicated. Simple carbohydrates, like sugar and candy, give the body an immediate energy boost by being quickly metabolized and absorbed. Whole grains and vegetables, which include complex carbs, are broken down more gradually and offer a steady supply of energy.

Carbohydrate Types

Simple Carbohydrates

Monosaccharides and disaccharides are examples of simple sugars, commonly referred to as simple carbohydrates. Single sugars include glucose and fructose, while disaccharides combine two sugars to form sucrose (table sugar) and lactose (milk sugar).

Sugary foods and beverages including candy, soda, and fruit juice frequently contain simple carbs.

Complex Carbohydrates

Polysaccharides, another name for complex carbohydrates, are composed of extended chains of sugar molecules. They include fiber, which is included in foods like vegetables, fruits, and whole grains, as well as starch, which is present in foods like bread, pasta, and rice. Complex carbs release energy more gradually and over a longer period of time than simple carbohydrates.

How Carbohydrates Affect Losing Weight

Because they give the body energy, carbohydrates aid in weight loss by boosting metabolism and enabling physical exercise. But taking an excessive amount of carbs, especially simple carbohydrates, might result in weight gain. This is due to the fact that simple carbs can cause blood sugar levels to rise quickly, which can boost the production of insulin and cause fat storage.

Contrarily, complex carbs offer a slower, more prolonged release of energy, which helps to regulate appetite and avoid overeating. Additionally, fiber, a form of complex carbohydrate, promotes weight loss by prolonging satiety by slowing digestion.

A healthy diet should generally contain a balance of both simple and complex carbs, with a focus on the latter. Choosing carbs from wholesome, nutritious sources, such as fruits, vegetables, and whole grains, rather than processed foods, and being mindful of portion sizes is also important.

In conclusion, carbohydrates are crucial for weight loss and ought to be a part of a healthy diet. Understanding the various forms of carbs and how they affect the body can help you make decisions that will help you achieve your weight loss objectives.

Chapter Three

How to Begin a Low-Carb Diet to Lose Weight

Choosing a Limit for Carbohydrates

Finding your daily carbohydrate limit is the first step in beginning a low-carb diet for weight loss. Numerous variables, such as your age, height, weight, and amount of physical activity, affect this figure. A low-carbohydrate diet typically caps daily carbohydrate intake at 20 to 50 grams.

You can consult a trained dietitian or nutritionist to determine your limit. They can assist you in figuring out how many calories you need to consume each day as well as how many carbohydrates you need to consume to meet those demands.

It's crucial to adhere to your carbohydrate restriction as precisely as you can once you've decided on one. This entails keeping track of how many grams of carbohydrates you eat at each meal and snack. To track your food intake and keep an eye on your carbohydrate intake, you can also utilize tools like a food journal or an app.

What to Eat If You're on a Low-Carb Diet

It's crucial to make the appropriate meal selections if you want to succeed with a low-carb diet. You must incorporate the following foods into your diet:

Meat and poultry: Meats such as chicken, beef, pork, and others are high in protein and low in carbs.

Shrimp, fish, and other seafood are all high in protein and low in carbs.

Eggs: Eggs are a fantastic source of protein and good fats. They also have a low carbohydrate content.

Dairy: Dairy products such as cheese, butter, and heavy cream are low in carbs and high in beneficial fats.

Nuts and seeds: Almonds, walnuts, sunflower seeds, and other nuts and seeds are nutritious sources of protein and healthy fats with little to no carbohydrate content.

Leafy greens, broccoli, cauliflower, and other vegetables are abundant in fiber, vitamins, and minerals yet low in carbs.

foods to avoid when following a low-carb diet

Avoiding certain foods that are high in carbohydrates will help you stay under your daily carbohydrate allowance. On a low-carbohydrate diet, you should stay away from the following foods:

Soft drinks, fruit juices, and other sugary beverages should be avoided because they are high in carbs.

Candy, cookies, and other sweets should be consumed in moderation because they are high in carbs.

Potatoes, rice, pasta, and other starchy foods should all be consumed in moderation because they are high in carbs.

Fruits high in carbohydrates: Fruits with a high carbohydrate content should be avoided, such as bananas, grapes, and mangoes.

Grains: Products made from grains, such as bread, cereal, and other baked goods, should be consumed in moderation.

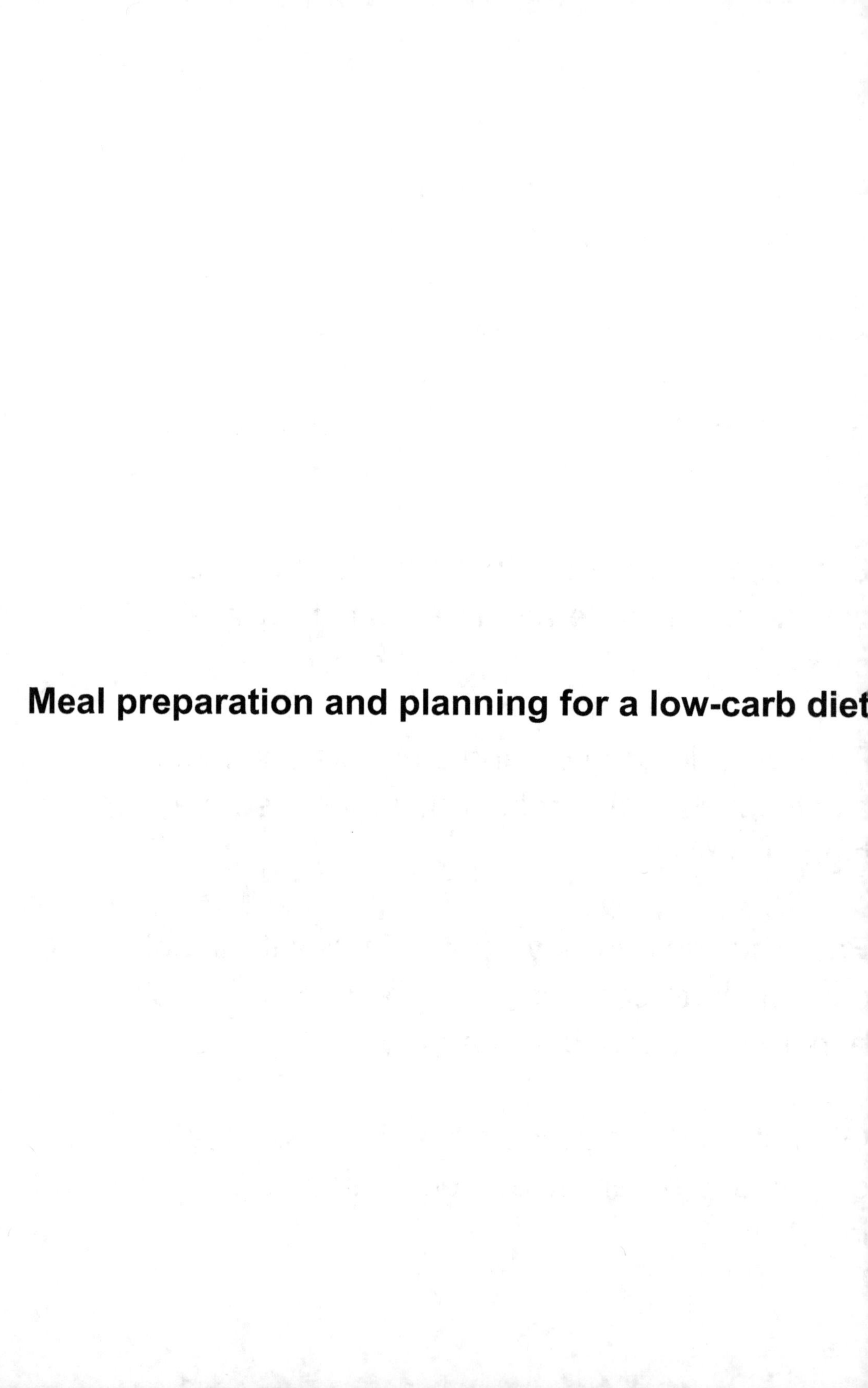

Meal preparation and planning for a low-carb diet

On a low-carb diet, meal preparation and planning are essential for success. Here are some pointers to get you going:

Take some time to plan your meals for the coming week. You can keep organized and make sure you're consuming the appropriate things in the right amounts thanks to this.

Make a list of the ingredients you'll need for your meals and snacks before you start shopping. Avoid buying high-carbohydrate items and stock up on low-carbohydrate alternatives instead.

Make your food: Making your food gives you control over the ingredients and ensures that you're eating low-carbohydrate items.

Bring your snacks: By bringing your snacks to work or when traveling, you may stay on your low-carb diet and avoid high-carb options. Hard-boiled eggs, nuts, seeds, and cheese make for tasty snacks.

Try fresh, innovative meals that are high in protein and healthy fats and low in carbohydrates. Try out new dishes to keep your diet interesting. There are plenty of delectable low-carb recipes online.

You can succeed on a low-carbohydrate diet for weight loss by adhering to these suggestions and using low-carbohydrate foods in your diet. Always pay attention to your body and make adjustments as necessary. If you require additional support, consult a registered dietitian or nutritionist.

Chapter Four

Building a Support Network

On a low-carbohydrate diet, it might be difficult to stay motivated. It necessitates commitment, resolve, and discipline. However, anyone can effectively follow this diet and achieve their weight reduction and health objectives with the correct attitude, resources, and support network. This book offers helpful advice and direction to keep you inspired as you pursue a low-carb diet.

It's important to have a solid support system when following a low-carbohydrate diet. Your support network can assist you in maintaining responsibility, motivation, and encouragement when things go tough. Here are a few strategies for building a helpful network:

Join a Low Carbohydrate Diet Community: Low Carbohydrate Diet communities can be found both online and offline. You can find a helpful atmosphere where you can share your experiences, ask questions, and receive support from others by joining these groups.

Find a Low-Carb Diet Buddy: It might be quite beneficial to have a friend or family member who is also on a low-carbohydrate diet. You can support one another and hold one another responsible.

Hire a Coach or Consultant: You might want to hire a coach or consultant if you need more support and direction. They can offer you individualized guidance and support to keep you inspired and on course.

Locating Recipes and Alternative Foods

Finding meals that adhere to your dietary requirements is one of the most difficult aspects of a low-carbohydrate diet. There are numerous substitute foods and recipes that are mouthwatering and low in carbs, though. Here are some pointers for locating substitute ingredients and recipes:

Try New Items: Experiment with new ingredients that are low in carbs, such as zucchini noodles, almond flour, and coconut flour.

Get Creative in the Kitchen: To make low-carbohydrate foods taste wonderful, experiment with different cooking techniques like grilling, baking, or roasting.

Utilize Recipe Books and Websites: There are numerous cookbooks and websites that are devoted to low-carbohydrate diets. Find new, delicious dishes that adhere to your dietary limitations using these resources.

Making Physical Activity a Regular Part of Your Life

Exercise is a crucial component of any weight loss plan, especially one that includes a low-carbohydrate diet. Exercise not only aids in calorie burning but also enhances general health and well-being. Here are some pointers for fitting exercise into your schedule:

Set Realistic Goals: Begin small and make sure your objectives are attainable. Consider setting a goal to work out for 30 minutes per day, three days per week.

Find a Sport You Like: Opt for a sport you like, like dancing, hiking, or swimming. You can maintain your schedule with the aid of this.

Make Exercise a Priority: Schedule regular exercise into your daily schedule to make it a priority in your life. You will be more motivated and responsible as a result.

Overcoming Stalls and Failures

Every effort to lose weight comes with difficulties and setbacks. Although plateaus and setbacks are common, it's crucial to have a strategy in place to go over them. Here are some pointers for getting beyond plateaus and obstacles:

Re-examine Your Food: If you've had a plateau, review your diet carefully to ensure that you're not over your carbohydrate allotment.

Consider boosting your level of physical exercise to speed up your metabolism and break through a plateau.

Even in the face of setbacks, it's critical to maintain optimism and focus on your goals. surround yourself with encouraging people and remember why you began your low.

Chapter Five

Typical errors that can impede your success

As with any diet, several typical blunders might impede your progress on a low-carb diet, which can be an efficient approach to losing weight and enhancing general health. In this book, we will look at some of the most typical low-carb diet errors and provide helpful advice on how to prevent them.

Avoiding Meals

When attempting to reduce your intake of carbohydrates, skipping meals can be appealing, but it can also be harmful. It is challenging to lose weight when you skip meals because your body enters "starvation mode" and starts to hang onto fat. Furthermore, missing meals might result in binge eating later in the day, which will quickly halt your progress.

It's crucial to eat regular, balanced meals throughout the day to prevent making this error. This will support you in maintaining a steady level of energy and a healthy metabolism. Avoid processed snacks and high-carbohydrate foods, and make an effort to include a source of protein, healthy fats, and veggies in each meal.

Overconsumption of processed foods

When attempting to reduce your carbohydrate intake, processed meals might be seductive, but they frequently contain artificial additives and bad fats. Even though they are low in carbohydrates, these foods can hinder your efforts and make it more difficult to lose weight.

Focus on consuming as many complete, unadulterated foods as you can to avoid making this error. Lean proteins, fresh fruits and vegetables, and nutritious fats like avocado and olive oil are all included in this. If you do eat processed foods, try to choose items that are prepared with mostly natural components and little sugar or preservative addition.

Getting Insufficient Water

On a low-carbohydrate diet, staying hydrated is very vital for overall health and weight loss. Dehydration can result in headaches, fatigue, and other unpleasant symptoms. The body needs water to process the extra ketones produced when you're in ketosis.

Make careful you have enough water during the day to prevent making this error. Aim for 8 glasses a day minimum, and up to more if you're working out or perspiring. To help you stay hydrated, you can also sip on herbal teas, unsweetened coconut water, or sparkling water.

Limiting your carbohydrate intake too strictly

While cutting back on carbohydrates is a crucial component of a low-carbohydrate diet, it's also necessary to be adaptable and give yourself some leeway. Being overly restrictive with your carbohydrate intake might result in cravings, binge eating, and exhaustion, which makes it more difficult to maintain your diet over the long term.

Try to be careful of your carbohydrate consumption without being unduly restrictive to avoid making this error. Give yourself the odd treat or higher-carb meal, and concentrate on overall balance rather than rigid adherence to a specific amount. Develop a low-carb diet plan that is nutritious and sustainable by consulting a dietitian or nutritionist.

You may maximize the benefits of your low-carbohydrate diet and reach your weight loss and health objectives by avoiding these frequent blunders. You'll be well on your road to success if you keep in mind to be persistent, patient, and balanced overall.

Chapter Six

How to Control Cravings and Hunger on a Low-Carb Diet

Anyone eating a low-carbohydrate diet may find it difficult to control their appetite and cravings. It is feasible to stick to your diet and achieve your goals, though, with a few straightforward methods and lifestyle adjustments. The detailed instructions in this book will show you how to control cravings and hunger while maintaining a low-carbohydrate diet.

Choosing Low-Carbohydrate Snacks:

It can be challenging to break the habit of snacking, especially when on a low-carbohydrate diet. However, it is feasible to locate scrumptious and gratifying low-carbohydrate snacks with a little imagination. Several possibilities are:

Raw seeds and nuts
Meats and cheese
vegetables such as cherry tomatoes, cucumbers, and carrots
Greek yogurt and fruit
Uncooked eggs
Additionally, it's critical to prepare ahead of time and keep low-carbohydrate snacks close at hand. When you have a stock of these snacks in your office, workout bag, or pantry, you'll be less likely to grab high-carbohydrate munchies.

Water Consumption and Hydration:

Keeping hydrated is crucial for controlling hunger and cravings. Drinking water might fill you up and keep you from overeating. Furthermore, dehydration can frequently be confused with hunger, so drinking plenty of water can prevent you from indulging in pointless food. Aim to consume at least 8 glasses of water each day, and think about keeping a water bottle with you at all times.

Participating in Physical Activity:

A wonderful technique to control cravings and hunger is exercise. Exercise can improve feelings of fullness and reduce stress. Exercise can also assist boost energy levels and elevate mood in general. It is advised to get at least 30 minutes of exercise every day, whether it be through a formal workout program or straightforward pursuits like riding, hiking, or strolling.

Alternative Stress-Reduction Techniques:

Stress frequently sets to cravings and binge eating. Reducing stress and preventing overeating can both be accomplished by finding other coping mechanisms. Among the techniques for reducing stress are:

Practices of mindfulness and meditation
Exercises for deep breathing
stretching and yoga
spending time in nature and being outside
taking part in hobbies and artistic pursuits

Conclusion:

A low-carb diet can make it difficult to control cravings and hunger, but by making a few little lifestyle adjustments, you can maintain your diet and achieve your objectives. Reduce cravings and avoid overeating by snacking on low-carbohydrate foods, staying hydrated, exercising, and finding alternative methods to cope with stress. You can successfully control cravings and hunger while maintaining a low-carb diet with a little perseverance.

Chapter Seven

How to Continue Losing Weight While Eating Few Carbs

For many people, losing weight and keeping it off can be difficult. Low-carbohydrate diets have gained popularity as a weight-loss option, but many people have trouble keeping their results over the long haul. This book is meant to serve as a resource for those who have successfully lost weight on a low-carbohydrate diet and are now looking for advice on how to keep it off and avoid gaining it back.

Reintroducing carbohydrates to your diet gradually

The progressive reintroduction of carbohydrates into your diet is one of the secrets to maintaining weight loss while following a low-carbohydrate diet. Your body may have adapted to utilize fat as its primary fuel source if you've been on a rigorous low-carb diet. Your body could have trouble adjusting if you abruptly up your carbohydrate intake, and you might put on weight as a result.

It's critical to gradually increase your carbohydrate intake over a few weeks to prevent this. Start by reintroducing tiny portions of low-carbohydrate foods to your diet, like whole grains, veggies, and fruit. You can add additional carbohydrates gradually until you achieve your preferred dietary level as your body adjusts.

Developing Stable Healthy Routines

On a low-carbohydrate diet, maintaining weight loss needs a long-term dedication to good behaviors. This entails following a balanced diet that is high in protein, fiber, and healthy fats while being low in carbohydrates. Additionally, it entails remaining active, exercising frequently, and abstaining from bad behaviors like binge drinking, smoking, and overeating.

Try to implement tiny, manageable adjustments, such as increasing your water intake, increasing your intake of fruits and vegetables, and reducing your portion sizes, to help you develop healthy habits. These modest adjustments over time might have significant effects, assisting you in maintaining your weight loss and leading a healthier lifestyle.

Maintaining Your Low Carbohydrate Lifestyle Through Exercise and Engagement

Another element of maintaining weight reduction success is continuing your low-carbohydrate lifestyle while remaining active. Maintaining your weight and enhancing your general health are both possible with regular exercise. Finding an activity you enjoy and sticking with it is crucial, whether you prefer to join in organized sports or prefer solo hobbies like walking, riding, or swimming.

It's crucial to continue living a low-carb lifestyle in addition to exercising. Connecting with people who have similar interests to yours, joining support groups, or taking part in online discussion forums or social media groups devoted to low-carbohydrate diets are some examples of how to do this.

Seeking Assistance and Direction When Needed

Finally, it's critical to get help and direction as needed when keeping weight off while following a low-carbohydrate diet. If you have any health problems, this may entail consulting a doctor or a dietitian who specializes in nutrition.

In conclusion, it takes a combination of good routines, consistent exercise, and social support to maintain weight loss on a low-carbohydrate diet. You can keep off the weight you've lost and have a better life by adhering to these recommendations and getting assistance when you need it.

Conclusion

In conclusion, studies have shown that low-carb diets are an efficient way to lose weight. By restricting the amount of carbs consumed, the body is compelled to use fat reserves as an energy source, which lowers body fat and promotes weight loss. Low-carb diets have also been demonstrated to enhance several health indicators, including cholesterol levels, blood sugar regulation, and insulin sensitivity.

Not all low-carbohydrate diets are made equal, and some may be more restrictive than others, it is crucial to remember this. It's also crucial to choose whole foods that are abundant in nutrients as opposed to processed foods that are heavy in calories as sources of carbohydrates. Additionally, it is critical to seek medical advice before beginning a low-carb diet, particularly for people with pre-existing medical concerns.

Overall, many people may find the low-carb strategy for weight loss to be a secure and reliable choice. People can successfully incorporate a low carbohydrate diet into their weight loss journey by making informed decisions and getting advice from a healthcare practitioner.

www.ingramcontent.com/pod-product-compliance
Lightning Source LLC
Chambersburg PA
CBHW051718250726
48653CB00008B/3098